STOP THE FAT, START THE FIT:

BE YOUR OWN PERSONAL TRAINER

BY BSTARR

DISCLAIMER

This book does not provide medical advice.
Results May Vary: Causes for being overweight or obese vary from person to person. Whether genetic or environmental, it should be noted that food intake, rates of metabolism and levels of exercise and physical exertion vary from person to person. This means weight loss results will also vary from person to person. No individual result should be seen as typical. These statements have not been evaluated by the Food and Drug Administration. This book is not intended to diagnose, treat, cure or prevent any disease.

The information, including but not limited to, text, graphics, images and other material, contained in this book is for personal purposes only. The content is not intended in any way as a substitute for professional medical advice, diagnosis or treatment. Always seek the advice of your physician or other qualified health care provider with any questions you may have regarding a medical condition or treatment and before undertaking a new health care regimen, and never disregard professional medical advice or delay in seeking it because of something you have read in this book.

SPECIAL THANKS

To my mother Deborah Starr, grandmother Bertha Wells, and uncle Tyrone VanHoesen. Thank you for having my back always and forever, no matter what. You all have supported me in everything I set out to do...whether you like it or not. You all are very appreciated.

To Anthony Stewart for giving me the idea to write this book. Without him, YOU would not be reading this. Anthony gave me the courage to write a book on something that I was not only embarassed about but also I did not think it was something special. He showed me just how important my weight loss journey was and how it could help others that were in my position as well.

To the rest of my family and friends. You also have supported me and helped me on this crazy rollercoaster called life. Without you, I wouldn't have been able to lose the weight and remake myself to be the best that I can be. Your encouragement, compliments, and enthusiam with me through my journey, not only with my weight loss but with my music as well is greatly appreciated.

DEDICATION

This book is for anyone out there who has ever had any negative feelings and/or thoughts about their appearance. This is for anyone who has endured any health complications due to being overweight. This is for those who have been bullied, teased, or mistreated in any other way because of their size or shape. This book is for the girls and boys, women and men, who are young and old that want to change their lives around. For those of us who are lost in the clouds...we are now found.

Chapter 1
THE FAT KID

At around the age of 5, I began to develop weight issues. My mother and grandmother always placed a lot of value on food. If I had a bad day at school my mother or grandmother would immediately either fix me something to eat or stop by my favorite fast food place. If I was feeling tired, they thought it was because I needed something to eat. This was even if I had just consumed a full meal only an hour or so before hand. If I was really happy about something, we would celebrate by eating my favorite meal. If I was in a bad mood it was due to the fact that I needed to eat. When we were out running errands all day it was mandatory to stop at a fast food restaurant because in their minds, I needed food to refuel me.

My mother and grandmother centered almost everything around food when it came to me for some odd reason. As an impressionable child, I started to keep this bad habit up on my own. I always felt the need to put something in my mouth whether I was hungry or not. There were even a lot of times where I'd eat just because I felt like I had nothing else to do. It was like an addiction. I would never even get full! What made my excessive eating worse was that most people around me didn't see an issue with it or my weight. Every now and then someone would make a snide remark but other than that, no one really bothered me about it. Family and friends were basically enablers.

As a kid, everyone just thought my being chubby was cute, and that it was baby fat that I'd lose or grow out of eventually. There were those kids though who did point it out from time to time. I will never forget the time when I was in the 4th grade. I was at afterschool care. Now I've always been a very opinionated and outspoken person so I guess you could say I had this coming. There was this little Caucasian boy in my class that was really short and picked his nose a lot. Over time I started making fun of him.

Usually, he just kind of ignored me when I made my rude comments, but this one particular time he retaliated. His response to my making fun of him was, "Well that's why you're fat!" He then proceeded to gather his friends to sing this little song about me. I will never forget the song because I was always a very strong individual when it came to grade school banter, but the teasing about my weight really hurt me. They sang "Fatty, Fatty, 2 by 4 can't even fit through the kitchen door...get it? KITCHEN DOOR!?" They laughed hysterically and made a big scene. To make matters worse, he and his other little friends also proceeded to tell me that I'd never be a star because I was too fat. My dream since I was a little girl was to become a singer/songwriter and actress. I used to tell all my schoolmates that they would see me on TV one day. Those little boys telling me that I wouldn't make it because I was fat crushed me.

From that day on I started to see my weight as a problem, but as a child, I still didn't know what to do to fix it. I just kept doing what I was used to. I proceeded to do what unfortunately came natural to me. Not to mention my closest friends were fat too so it was hard to try and change when everyone around me was going through and constantly doing the same thing. I never told anyone until this now how badly that boy and his friends hurt my feelings. I cried myself to sleep many nights just thinking about that day and how humiliated I felt. From that point, my self-esteem was at an all-time low and continued to plummet even further later on in my life.

Chapter 2
LAZY LIFE

From 4th grade all the way up until I was a sopho-more in high school, I was an extreme gamer and I also loved watching television. My mother was very overprotective of me so I was not allowed to go out-side and play very much like other kids. As a matter of fact, she would make sure that she purchased my favorite movie and video games, along with my favor-ite candy and/or food to snack on so that I wouldn't even want to go out and play. She did have a good reason though. The neighborhood we were in around that point and time of my life was not the safest so she was just trying to look out for me. On top of the latter, I also wasn't very active outside of gym class at school either. I did play sports off and on, but a game and practice maybe twice a week doesn't compare to eat-ing all kinds of fatty foods all throughout the day on a daily basis. Being a couch potato outside of school led me even further into a downward spiral with my weight.

My daily schedule at this time was school from 8am-3pm with an unhealthy breakfast in the morning. The breakfast was followed by an unhealthy snack in be-tween that time and lunch. The lunch was unhealthy as well and along with me having a bottomless pit for a stomach, I also had seconds and sometimes even thirds.

After school, due to my mother having to work until 5pm or 6pm every day, I attended after school care. There, again, I was presented with more fatty foods and snacks until my mother came to pick me up. When we got home, I'd have another snack until dinner was ready. I would then eat dinner while playing my video games or watching TV. After dinner, I was pretty much gaming, watching TV, and eating all throughout the night until I went to sleep. This horrible regimen was followed every day and got even worse on the weekends.

I would spend most Saturdays and Sundays in front of the TV with food and snacks all throughout the day. After I did my homework, the remainder of the day involved little to no physical activity whatsoever. My idea of a great weekend consisted of all the food and snacks I wanted paired with action and comedy movies like 007, Denzel Washington movies, Shrek, and Zoolander just to name a few. One of my favorite games to play at the time was The Sims, and Grand Theft Auto on PlayStation. Basically, from my adolescent years up to my teens, I was nothing but a couch potato with very out of control eating habits. By the time I was in 7th grade all the way to Freshman year of high school, my weight would fluctuate between 175 to 190lbs.

Chapter 3
AT A LOSS

You would think that by the time I hit age 15 and was in high school that my "baby fat" would have left me right? WRONG! The cute chubby kid then turned into the ugly, fat teen. As a teen entering high school you would think that I would have gotten teased and picked on about my weight. Surprisingly, no one paid much attention to my weight, which still made me feel kind of like it wasn't too much of an issue. On the other hand, I knew something was wrong because I didn't feel good. Being fat also made it difficult to look in the mirror. I thought I was really ugly, so my self-esteem was nonexistent by then. At 15, I weighed about 188lbs. When I hit age 17, I got my first boyfriend! Also, miraculously, about a year after I met my first boyfriend I lost 44lbs without even trying! I weighed the least I think I have ever weighed in my life! What triggered it was me wanting to look as good as possible for my new boyfriend paired with hanging out with friends instead of sitting in front of the TV like I used to. Another reason the weight came off really quickly was because I joined the dance line team. I was much more active.

Our coach worked us like we were in boot camp. We met to do extreme workouts about 4 times a week and these were grueling, but obviously worked. Dance line was short lived due to financial reasons. Then in addition to having to quit dance line, I was forced to go on birth control since I had a boyfriend and was now sexually active. The first method I tried was the Depo-Provera birth control. This was administered as a shot that I got from my doctor every three months. This is when I was around 18, and my weight issues came back in full force.

Every three months when I would go to get the shot, I was always 15-20lbs heavier than the last visit. By the end of my senior year in high school, I was 235lbs. I knew that it was time for something to change. I got my contraceptive switched to the pill which isn't as harmful and has less hormonal effects than the Depo-Provera shots. However, I then noticed that while the pills were not making me gain weight, they weren't allowing me to lose weight either. I started working out and sometimes starving myself, and my weight never changed. Around that time, I was 19 going on 20. My boyfriend, family, and friends didn't notice but I was seriously starting to have major complications from being overweight. Any little bit of activity I did would make me feel like I was going to faint or have a heart attack. Doing the laundry would have me out of breath and feeling exhausted just after one trip up and down the stairs. Doing things like walking around at the park or zoo would make my ankles hurt really badly, and leave me feeling very faint. I didn't even enjoy sex anymore. Every time he and I were intimate, my heart felt like it was going to burst. I tried my best to hide it, but every time I had sex, I felt like I was dying. By the time I was nearing 21, I decided that I had ENOUGH!

 I went to my doctor to see if there was a medical issue. When she weighed me, the scale read 245 lbs. I was terribly overweight, especially for my height of only 5 feet tall. By medical standards, at 5ft tall I should only weigh at the most 130lbs. My doctor ran tests, and everything surprisingly came back fine. She did state, however, that my metabolism was very slow and that I could change all of that with diet and exercise. To jumpstart my weight loss, she put me on a weight loss pill. I lost 25lbs in three weeks. After I lost the first 25lbs, she took me off of it because it is harmful if used for long periods of time. Also, she wanted me to lose it naturally because obviously that is the healthier way and holds more longevity. I started back working out at home, but that became hard for me to do. I was the only fat person trying to lose weight in my household so it was kind of hard to run in place and do crunches while people were walking around eating ice cream bars, cakes, and candies. At home, I just felt like I wasn't being encouraged enough and needed a better atmosphere. At 220lbs, I decided to enroll myself in a gym. I chose a gym located close to home mostly due to the affordability and convenience. Joining this gym along with making extreme changes to my diet started my journey to losing weight.

Chapter 4
YOU ARE HOW YOU EAT

You wanted to know my big weight loss "secret" so here we go! Diet is the most important part of losing weight. I repeat, DIET IS THE MOST IMPORTANT PART OF LOSING WEIGHT! I've been able to lose 15-20lbs without even touching the gym. Your eating habits control almost everything. The way you eat can control your energy, your health, your mind, and your body. Everything you put in your mouth has either a negative, positive, or neutral effect on your body. For example, the coffee bean is a natural metabolism booster. If you are a coffee drinker, especially if you drink it black (meaning no added sugars or other artificial flavoring), this will give you more energy, and allow you to lose more weight and burn calories at a faster rate. My previous diet consisted of whatever I wanted whenever I wanted it. Sometimes I was eating 6 or 7 times a day. I had 3 main meals along with 4 other little meals and/or very unhealthy snacks. This was every day. This is the diet that led me to being almost 300lbs.

We are really only supposed to eat to live, not live to eat. This means that instead of eating simply because it makes you feel good or because it tastes good, you should eat only because you have to in order to properly function on a daily basis. As an overweight person, your stomach is basically stretched out. This means that you are able to consume a very large amount of food, and it will also take longer to get full. I started to watch what I ate along with counting calories. I would try my best to make sure I only ate 1500 calories a day. The easiest way to make sure I didn't go over 1500 calories was to eat things that I knew weren't high in calories such as a small bowl of cereal for breakfast, a salad for lunch, and another salad or a grilled chicken breast along with some spinach for dinner. If I get hungry in between those meals, I'd eat a piece of fruit and/or drink a bottle of water. I'd keep up this routine for a while then gradually decrease my caloric intake. I now make sure I only eat 1200 calories per day.

Also keep in mind that our bodies don't really need all of the food that doctors and nutritionists say we need. There is absolutely nothing wrong with eating only once a day or even skipping eating on some days all together. If you think about it, food is a business so it only makes sense to tell people that they need to eat around the clock in order to benefit sales. We are only told to eat breakfast, lunch, dinner, and small snacks in between, so that BIG BUSINESS can make their profit. Eating around the clock is very unhealthy. This is because it actually takes our bodies a full 24 hours to fully and successfully digest one basic meal (you can google "24hrs to digest a meal" and you'll find the information on it is accurate). So when you eat several different snacks and meals throughout the day, you are throwing your body's natural healing and functioning abilities off course. This is also what leads to different illnesses and can cause our bodies to become weak and broken down over time.

I eat what I want to eat. For example, I try my best to stay away from cheeseburgers, but every now and then I honestly just can't help but to grab a juicy, greasy, mouthwatering burger! Even though now I eat turkey burgers because I no longer eat beef or pork. To make matters even worse, I go ahead and eat the fries too, and get my favorite shake to add to this caloric chaos! At this point, you are probably thinking, "This woman is mad! There's no way she lost 90lbs eating like that!" WRONG! It is ok to eat the way you want to without any restrictions as long as you make sure it doesn't become a habit. Cheat days are a MUST HAVE when trying to lose weight. This is because you cannot possibly go from eating like crazy to barely eating anything ever and be able to maintain that diet long term. You will eventually go on a huge binge-eating spree, and before you know it you'll be 10lbs heavier in just a week.
You have to be able to still eat and drink your favorite things. I usually use some Fridays as my cheat days. I allow myself two cheat days per month and if I have more than two, I make sure I burn the calories off by hitting the gym much harder than usual. My diet is all about balance. If I over eat, I over exercise. If I skipped a day of eating or have a good day where

I only eat 800-1200 calories, I can skip the gym or just have a slight workout. To sum everything up, EAT AND DRINK WHATEVER YOU WANT in moderation. The more you eat the more you should exercise, but the smaller the portion the better. Caffeine is you best friend, and DO NOT EAT MUCH AFTER 6PM.

Chapter 5
A POUND LIGHTER, FASTER

With my new eating habits, I was definitely seeing results. I enrolled at a local gym and purchased the $20.00 per month membership so that I had full access to the gym 24/7 along with the perks of being able to try out different classes. I tried spin, yoga, turbo kick, body pump, and pretty much every class except for Zumba Fitness. For some reason, I was a bit reluctant to try it, partly because it didn't look like it was high impact enough. The workouts that burn the most calories, around 500-1000, are usually the ones that are very high impact. You know, the ones where afterwards you're drenched in sweat and literally wet from head to toe. One day, a friend of mine suggested that I try it. After constantly complaining about how I'd probably suck at it and saying that it didn't look like it was for me, I finally went ahead and tried it.

I then found my true calling! I fell in love with Zumba Fitness! Zumba Fitness is a Latin-dance inspired workout. I also saw even more dramatic results while eating right and constantly doing Zumba workouts. I did this Zumba routine about two times a week along with going to the gym regularly three times a week. I made sure that between Zumba and my regular workouts I was being active at least five times a week. This made losing weight even easier because since I wasn't eating much along with burning lots of calories, I was losing up to 2lbs per day! The reason why Zumba Fitness is so fun and popular is because it leaves room for interpretation. Zumba does not require lots of intricate dance steps which can be frustrating, especially for people who don't have much rhythm or aren't dancers. It is much better than an aerobics class because you can basically dance the way you want and you don't necessarily have to follow the instructor. Zumba is literally like going to a club to dance your butt off for an hour. I seriously encourage you to try it!

Chapter 6
MONDAY THROUGH SUNDAY WORKOUTS

Along with taking Zumba classes now at least once a week (due to my work schedule constantly changing at the time), I developed my own workout regimen. Mondays consists' of 30 minutes of running on the treadmill or using the elliptical for 30 minutes, an hour of Zumba, 100 squats, and 100 crunches. Tuesdays consists' of 30 minutes on the treadmill, 30 minutes on the elliptical, 100 squats, 100 lunges along with other leg workouts, and 100 crunches. Wednesdays consists' of 30 minutes on the elliptical, 30 minutes on the stair master, 100 squats, different arm workouts with 8-10 pound barbells, and 100 crunches. Thursdays are basically Tuesdays repeated. Fridays are basically Wednesdays repeated. Saturdays consists' of an hour of running either on a treadmill, at the park, or around the neighborhood, 100 squats, and 100 crunches. Sundays consists' of simply a 1 hour run along with 100 squats. I try to use Sundays as a rest day but still want to get a slight workout in.

I repeated this routine every day for months when I first started out. Of course, some days got skipped because life does happen. As long as you stay on this course as much as possible and make up for the lost day, you will continue to see great results. Notice how

I make sure I do at least 100 squats per day. This is because unfortunately most of my weight is in my hips, butt, and thighs. Squats not only keep the butt firm and toned, but they also make your hips and thighs look toned too. Having more weight on the lower portion of your body can allow for unsightly cellulite. The more squats and leg work you do, the less cellulite you will see.

Chapter 7
GET ADDICTED TO HOW YOU LOOK

I used to hate mirrors. I did not like looking in them, walking past them, or even just having one around. Being fat over the years gave me immense image issues. I was constantly depressed and sad. I felt inadequate, disgusting, gross, and even wanted to die. I would spend lots of time wondering why I was even here on this Earth. Who would create such a waste like me? I felt so fat and ugly to the point of agony. But that was then. I seriously started my weight loss journey in the year of 2010 at 240lbs. and by the time the year of 2012 rolled around I was 150lbs. I lost a total of 90lbs! I became addicted to my new look. My self-esteem skyrocketed, and I was the happiest I had ever been in my life. For the first time in a very long time, I finally felt like a normal person. I could walk out of the house with my head held high. I could hold wonderful conversations with people, go to events, mingle, and feel confident the entire time.

I was no longer scared to be around people or to go out in public. Everywhere I went I was getting lots of compliments and attention. I finally overcame the one thing that was holding me back all of my life, FAT. The new and improved me now loves mirrors. In fact, I can't keep out of them, especially full length mirrors. I am now even doing things I never thought I'd do. I am following my dream of being a singer/songwriter. This is something I've always wanted to do but when you are stuck and in complete darkness in your life, dreams seem so far away and unattainable. I have been performing all over St. Louis, MO, have an album on the way, workout classes beginning, and still many more things to come. However, the battle is still in progress. At now 150 pounds, I am still on a mission to lose at least 30 more pounds.

Chapter 8
MAKEOVER

I went from a size 22 to my current pants size of a 9! I have finally made it to the single digits! This was the first time since I was maybe 13 years old being able to wear size small/medium tops and a size 9 in pants. For the first time in almost forever, I can go into department stores and not feel horrible about myself. I can shop in the regular sections instead of the plus size sections. I was finally able to say goodbye to plus size clothing stores. I can actually fit everything I want to buy and it feels so liberating. I decided since my body had a new hot look, I should re-invent myself entirely. I went and created what I call the new B! I am no longer self-conscious and a victim of low self-esteem. This made becoming the new, hot, better B easy.

I started my new look by changing my wardrobe. First of all, my wardrobe had to change anyway because since I lost so much weight, nothing could fit anymore. Secondly, I now have the confidence to start dressing for my age and body type. Before I lost weight, I would unfortunately make the mistake of making myself look even bigger by wearing huge tops and pants. I would also stay really covered up. To make matters worse, clothes that are for "plus size' women aren't really flattering and can also sometimes have more of an old fashioned look. I began buying clothes that fit my curves perfectly. I also started wearing heels for the first time. Back when I was fat, I couldn't wear heels because of carrying around so much weight. I also changed my hairstyle. I wore my hair in a very plain jane way for years. My hairstyle was long extensions day in and day out, 24/7, three hundred sixty-five days a year.

To go with my new hot body, I needed a new, hot style. I decided to cut my hair. This made me look even more fierce! I now have the body I NEVER thought I'd see, an edgy and hot hairstyle I would have NEVER dared to try, and I can now hold my head up high wherever I go!

Chapter 9
PLAY KEEP AWAY

Once you get to your happy place, as I have, you absolutely by all means CANNOT STOP THE ROUTINE. We have worked way too hard and have gone too far to let that fat creep back up on us. Once you see the results of your hard work, it is easy to get a bit lazy. Yes, we do need to reward ourselves with maybe a bit of a vacation, favorite food, pastime, etc., but we do not want to relax too hard or too long. Maintaining the new you is key because too many slip-ups can equal rising pounds, inches, and pant sizes. I stay focused mostly by looking at old photos from when I used to be fat. Keep a few of those horrible, fatty pictures of you around the house. I keep my FAT ASS pictures hung up on the wall right beside my mirror to remind me of how far I have come and how much I truly do not want to end up back there.

Stick to your workout routines and calorie counting. Look in the mirror every day and admire the hell out of yourself. I've also found it really helpful to set new challenges for myself. For example, even though I have gotten down to my target weight, I still see things that could use some additional work. I focus on those things, which helps keep me on top of my game. Also keep in mind it is ok to say NO. Sometimes we get invited to parties and other social events and some sort of desert, food, and/or liquor is provided. I know! I know! It is really hard to say no, especially to FREE FOOD and DRINKS! Don't let that deter you, and try to keep a record of what you have consumed throughout the day. I have a little thing I like to do especially when I know I will be partying or consuming liquor. Remember, this is MY WAY of losing weight and keeping if off; you do not have to follow this. I usually eat really light, such as one salad for the entire day, and drink only water until it is time to party. That way I basically substitute my calories so that I am not eating 1200-1500 calories on top of drinking about 1200 calories. Keeping a good record lets you know if you can afford to eat a little something extra or not.

Chapter 10
LOVE YOU, LIVE YOU

So now it is time. From this moment on, work on the new you. Transform yourself into that awesome, sexy, heart throb, girl or guy you have always wanted to be. Losing weight is not hard. What is hard is putting yourself and your mind in the positive state it needs to constantly be in to achieve your weight loss goal. Do not focus on other people and what they are doing or saying. This is now YOUR TIME. You may even have to take a break from certain friends, family, and activities, but trust me it is worth it. Some people will try to force their opinions on you, but smile and stay on YOUR PATH. Some will say, "You look fine the way you are!", but smile and STICK WITH IT. People will say, "Oh it's ok to just eat a little of the ice cream!", but smile and KINDLY DECLINE.

It will take time. You will struggle. There will be pain. You will cry. You will have set backs. You will "be hungry". Your body will go through several changes, but YOU WILL KEEP GOING; YOU MUST KEEP GOING. In the process of losing weight and becoming a better you, YOU MUST STAY POSITIVE no matter what. You may only lose a pound a week or maybe only 2 pounds in 2 weeks but guess what? LOSING is LOSING...PERIOD. Every loss, whether big or small, fast or slow is a GAIN towards your GOAL! The Universe loves you. I love you. Now it is time for you to LOVE YOU!

www.ingramcontent.com/pod-product-compliance
Lightning Source LLC
Chambersburg PA
CBHW071320280526
45788CB00004B/1958